AF824757

GET IT MADE.

THE ULTIMATE MEAL PLANNER
FOR GETTING MADE
WHAT NEEDS TO GET MADE

CoyoteCrest

Weekly Meal Plan for ____________________

	BREAKFAST	LUNCH	DINNER	SNACKS
S				
M				
T				
W				
T				
F				
S				

Weekly Groceries for ____________________

NOTES

Weekly Meal Plan for ______________________

	BREAKFAST	LUNCH	DINNER	SNACKS
S				
M				
T				
W				
T				
F				
S				

Weekly Groceries for ______________________

- [ ]
- [ ]
- [ ]
- [ ]
- [ ]
- [ ]
- [ ]
- [ ]
- [ ]
- [ ]
- [ ]
- [ ]
- [ ]
- [ ]
- [ ]
- [ ]
- [ ]
- [ ]
- [ ]
- [ ]
- [ ]
- [ ]
- [ ]

- [ ]
- [ ]
- [ ]
- [ ]
- [ ]
- [ ]
- [ ]
- [ ]
- [ ]
- [ ]
- [ ]
- [ ]
- [ ]
- [ ]
- [ ]
- [ ]
- [ ]
- [ ]
- [ ]
- [ ]
- [ ]
- [ ]
- [ ]

NOTES

Weekly Meal Plan for ____________________

	BREAKFAST	LUNCH	DINNER	SNACKS
S				
M				
T				
W				
T				
F				
S				

Weekly Groceries for ____________________

NOTES

Weekly Meal Plan for ________________

	BREAKFAST	LUNCH	DINNER	SNACKS
S				
M				
T				
W				
T				
F				
S				

Weekly Groceries for ______________________

NOTES

Weekly Meal Plan for ____________

	BREAKFAST	LUNCH	DINNER	SNACKS
S				
M				
T				
W				
T				
F				
S				

Weekly Groceries for ____________

NOTES

Weekly Meal Plan for ____________________

	BREAKFAST	LUNCH	DINNER	SNACKS
S				
M				
T				
W				
T				
F				
S				

Weekly Groceries for ______________________

NOTES

Weekly Meal Plan for ______________

	BREAKFAST	LUNCH	DINNER	SNACKS
S				
M				
T				
W				
T				
F				
S				

Weekly Groceries for ______________________

NOTES

Weekly Meal Plan for ______________________

	BREAKFAST	LUNCH	DINNER	SNACKS
S				
M				
T				
W				
T				
F				
S				

Weekly Groceries for ____________________

NOTES

Weekly Meal Plan for ____________________

	BREAKFAST	LUNCH	DINNER	SNACKS
S				
M				
T				
W				
T				
F				
S				

Weekly Groceries for ______________________

NOTES

Weekly Meal Plan for ____________________

	BREAKFAST	LUNCH	DINNER	SNACKS
S				
M				
T				
W				
T				
F				
S				

Weekly Groceries for ____________________

- [ ] ____________________
- [ ] ____________________
- [ ] ____________________
- [ ] ____________________
- [ ] ____________________
- [ ] ____________________
- [ ] ____________________
- [ ] ____________________
- [ ] ____________________
- [ ] ____________________
- [ ] ____________________
- [ ] ____________________
- [ ] ____________________
- [ ] ____________________
- [ ] ____________________
- [ ] ____________________
- [ ] ____________________
- [ ] ____________________
- [ ] ____________________
- [ ] ____________________
- [ ] ____________________
- [ ] ____________________
- [ ] ____________________

- [ ] ____________________
- [ ] ____________________
- [ ] ____________________
- [ ] ____________________
- [ ] ____________________
- [ ] ____________________
- [ ] ____________________
- [ ] ____________________
- [ ] ____________________
- [ ] ____________________
- [ ] ____________________
- [ ] ____________________
- [ ] ____________________
- [ ] ____________________
- [ ] ____________________
- [ ] ____________________
- [ ] ____________________
- [ ] ____________________
- [ ] ____________________
- [ ] ____________________
- [ ] ____________________
- [ ] ____________________
- [ ] ____________________

NOTES

Weekly Meal Plan for ____________________

	BREAKFAST	LUNCH	DINNER	SNACKS
S				
M				
T				
W				
T				
F				
S				

Weekly Groceries for ______________________

- [ ] ______________________
- [ ] ______________________
- [ ] ______________________
- [ ] ______________________
- [ ] ______________________
- [ ] ______________________
- [ ] ______________________
- [ ] ______________________
- [ ] ______________________
- [ ] ______________________
- [ ] ______________________
- [ ] ______________________
- [ ] ______________________
- [ ] ______________________
- [ ] ______________________
- [ ] ______________________
- [ ] ______________________
- [ ] ______________________
- [ ] ______________________
- [ ] ______________________
- [ ] ______________________
- [ ] ______________________
- [ ] ______________________
- [ ] ______________________
- [ ] ______________________
- [ ] ______________________
- [ ] ______________________
- [ ] ______________________
- [ ] ______________________
- [ ] ______________________
- [ ] ______________________
- [ ] ______________________
- [ ] ______________________
- [ ] ______________________
- [ ] ______________________
- [ ] ______________________
- [ ] ______________________
- [ ] ______________________
- [ ] ______________________
- [ ] ______________________
- [ ] ______________________
- [ ] ______________________
- [ ] ______________________
- [ ] ______________________
- [ ] ______________________
- [ ] ______________________

NOTES

Weekly Meal Plan for ____________________

	BREAKFAST	LUNCH	DINNER	SNACKS
S				
M				
T				
W				
T				
F				
S				

Weekly Groceries for ____________________

NOTES

Weekly Meal Plan for ____________________

	BREAKFAST	LUNCH	DINNER	SNACKS
S				
M				
T				
W				
T				
F				
S				

Weekly Groceries for ______________________

NOTES

Weekly Meal Plan for ____________________

	BREAKFAST	LUNCH	DINNER	SNACKS
S				
M				
T				
W				
T				
F				
S				

Weekly Groceries for ____________________

NOTES

Weekly Meal Plan for ____________________

	BREAKFAST	LUNCH	DINNER	SNACKS
S				
M				
T				
W				
T				
F				
S				

Weekly Groceries for ____________________

NOTES

Weekly Meal Plan for ____________________

	BREAKFAST	LUNCH	DINNER	SNACKS
S				
M				
T				
W				
T				
F				
S				

Weekly Groceries for ____________________

NOTES

Weekly Meal Plan for ____________________

	BREAKFAST	LUNCH	DINNER	SNACKS
S				
M				
T				
W				
T				
F				
S				

Weekly Groceries for ____________________

- [ ] ____________________
- [ ] ____________________
- [ ] ____________________
- [ ] ____________________
- [ ] ____________________
- [ ] ____________________
- [ ] ____________________
- [ ] ____________________
- [ ] ____________________
- [ ] ____________________
- [ ] ____________________
- [ ] ____________________
- [ ] ____________________
- [ ] ____________________
- [ ] ____________________
- [ ] ____________________
- [ ] ____________________
- [ ] ____________________
- [ ] ____________________
- [ ] ____________________
- [ ] ____________________
- [ ] ____________________
- [ ] ____________________

- [ ] ____________________
- [ ] ____________________
- [ ] ____________________
- [ ] ____________________
- [ ] ____________________
- [ ] ____________________
- [ ] ____________________
- [ ] ____________________
- [ ] ____________________
- [ ] ____________________
- [ ] ____________________
- [ ] ____________________
- [ ] ____________________
- [ ] ____________________
- [ ] ____________________
- [ ] ____________________
- [ ] ____________________
- [ ] ____________________
- [ ] ____________________
- [ ] ____________________
- [ ] ____________________
- [ ] ____________________
- [ ] ____________________

NOTES

Weekly Meal Plan for ____________________

	BREAKFAST	LUNCH	DINNER	SNACKS
S				
M				
T				
W				
T				
F				
S				

Weekly Groceries for ______________________

NOTES

Weekly Meal Plan for ____________________

	BREAKFAST	LUNCH	DINNER	SNACKS
S				
M				
T				
W				
T				
F				
S				

Weekly Groceries for ______________________

NOTES

Weekly Meal Plan for ____________________

	BREAKFAST	LUNCH	DINNER	SNACKS
S				
M				
T				
W				
T				
F				
S				

Weekly Groceries for ____________________

NOTES

Weekly Meal Plan for ____________________

	BREAKFAST	LUNCH	DINNER	SNACKS
S				
M				
T				
W				
T				
F				
S				

Weekly Groceries for ______________________

NOTES

Weekly Meal Plan for ____________________

	BREAKFAST	LUNCH	DINNER	SNACKS
S				
M				
T				
W				
T				
F				
S				

Weekly Groceries for ____________________

NOTES

Weekly Meal Plan for ________________

	BREAKFAST	LUNCH	DINNER	SNACKS
S				
M				
T				
W				
T				
F				
S				

Weekly Groceries for ______________________

NOTES

Weekly Meal Plan for ______________________

	BREAKFAST	LUNCH	DINNER	SNACKS
S				
M				
T				
W				
T				
F				
S				

Weekly Groceries for ______________________

NOTES

Weekly Meal Plan for ______________

	BREAKFAST	LUNCH	DINNER	SNACKS
S				
M				
T				
W				
T				
F				
S				

Weekly Groceries for ________________

NOTES

Weekly Meal Plan for ____________________

	BREAKFAST	LUNCH	DINNER	SNACKS
S				
M				
T				
W				
T				
F				
S				

Weekly Groceries for ____________________

NOTES

Weekly Meal Plan for ______________

	BREAKFAST	LUNCH	DINNER	SNACKS
S				
M				
T				
W				
T				
F				
S				

Weekly Groceries for ____________________

NOTES

Weekly Meal Plan for ______________________

	BREAKFAST	LUNCH	DINNER	SNACKS
S				
M				
T				
W				
T				
F				
S				

Weekly Groceries for ____________________

NOTES

Weekly Meal Plan for ____________________

	BREAKFAST	LUNCH	DINNER	SNACKS
S				
M				
T				
W				
T				
F				
S				

Weekly Groceries for ______________________

☐ ______________________ ☐ ______________________
☐ ______________________ ☐ ______________________
☐ ______________________ ☐ ______________________
☐ ______________________ ☐ ______________________
☐ ______________________ ☐ ______________________
☐ ______________________ ☐ ______________________
☐ ______________________ ☐ ______________________
☐ ______________________ ☐ ______________________
☐ ______________________ ☐ ______________________
☐ ______________________ ☐ ______________________
☐ ______________________ ☐ ______________________
☐ ______________________ ☐ ______________________
☐ ______________________ ☐ ______________________
☐ ______________________ ☐ ______________________
☐ ______________________ ☐ ______________________
☐ ______________________ ☐ ______________________
☐ ______________________ ☐ ______________________
☐ ______________________ ☐ ______________________
☐ ______________________ ☐ ______________________
☐ ______________________ ☐ ______________________
☐ ______________________ ☐ ______________________
☐ ______________________ ☐ ______________________
☐ ______________________ ☐ ______________________

NOTES

Weekly Meal Plan for ______________________

	BREAKFAST	LUNCH	DINNER	SNACKS
S				
M				
T				
W				
T				
F				
S				

Weekly Groceries for ________________________

- [ ] ____________________
- [ ] ____________________
- [ ] ____________________
- [ ] ____________________
- [ ] ____________________
- [ ] ____________________
- [ ] ____________________
- [ ] ____________________
- [ ] ____________________
- [ ] ____________________
- [ ] ____________________
- [ ] ____________________
- [ ] ____________________
- [ ] ____________________
- [ ] ____________________
- [ ] ____________________
- [ ] ____________________
- [ ] ____________________
- [ ] ____________________
- [ ] ____________________
- [ ] ____________________
- [ ] ____________________
- [ ] ____________________
- [ ] ____________________
- [ ] ____________________
- [ ] ____________________
- [ ] ____________________
- [ ] ____________________
- [ ] ____________________
- [ ] ____________________
- [ ] ____________________
- [ ] ____________________
- [ ] ____________________
- [ ] ____________________
- [ ] ____________________
- [ ] ____________________
- [ ] ____________________
- [ ] ____________________
- [ ] ____________________
- [ ] ____________________
- [ ] ____________________
- [ ] ____________________
- [ ] ____________________
- [ ] ____________________
- [ ] ____________________
- [ ] ____________________

NOTES

Weekly Meal Plan for ____________________

	BREAKFAST	LUNCH	DINNER	SNACKS
S				
M				
T				
W				
T				
F				
S				

Weekly Groceries for ____________________

- [ ] ____________________
- [ ] ____________________

NOTES

Weekly Meal Plan for ____________

	BREAKFAST	LUNCH	DINNER	SNACKS
S				
M				
T				
W				
T				
F				
S				

Weekly Groceries for ____________________

NOTES

Weekly Meal Plan for ____________________

	BREAKFAST	LUNCH	DINNER	SNACKS
S				
M				
T				
W				
T				
F				
S				

Weekly Groceries for ____________________

☐ ____________________ ☐ ____________________

NOTES

Weekly Meal Plan for ____________________

	BREAKFAST	LUNCH	DINNER	SNACKS
S				
M				
T				
W				
T				
F				
S				

Weekly Groceries for ____________________

NOTES

Weekly Meal Plan for ____________________

	BREAKFAST	LUNCH	DINNER	SNACKS
S				
M				
T				
W				
T				
F				
S				

Weekly Groceries for ______________________

☐ ______________________ ☐ ______________________

☐ ______________________ ☐ ______________________

☐ ______________________ ☐ ______________________

☐ ______________________ ☐ ______________________

☐ ______________________ ☐ ______________________

☐ ______________________ ☐ ______________________

☐ ______________________ ☐ ______________________

☐ ______________________ ☐ ______________________

☐ ______________________ ☐ ______________________

☐ ______________________ ☐ ______________________

☐ ______________________ ☐ ______________________

☐ ______________________ ☐ ______________________

☐ ______________________ ☐ ______________________

☐ ______________________ ☐ ______________________

☐ ______________________ ☐ ______________________

☐ ______________________ ☐ ______________________

☐ ______________________ ☐ ______________________

☐ ______________________ ☐ ______________________

☐ ______________________ ☐ ______________________

☐ ______________________ ☐ ______________________

☐ ______________________ ☐ ______________________

☐ ______________________ ☐ ______________________

☐ ______________________ ☐ ______________________

NOTES

Weekly Meal Plan for ____________________

	BREAKFAST	LUNCH	DINNER	SNACKS
S				
M				
T				
W				
T				
F				
S				

Weekly Groceries for ___________________

NOTES

Weekly Meal Plan for ____________

	BREAKFAST	LUNCH	DINNER	SNACKS
S				
M				
T				
W				
T				
F				
S				

Weekly Groceries for ______________________

NOTES

Weekly Meal Plan for ____________________

	BREAKFAST	LUNCH	DINNER	SNACKS
S				
M				
T				
W				
T				
F				
S				

Weekly Groceries for ______________________

NOTES

Weekly Meal Plan for ____________________

	BREAKFAST	LUNCH	DINNER	SNACKS
S				
M				
T				
W				
T				
F				
S				

Weekly Groceries for ______________________

- [ ] ____________________
- [ ] ____________________

NOTES

Weekly Meal Plan for ____________________

	BREAKFAST	LUNCH	DINNER	SNACKS
S				
M				
T				
W				
T				
F				
S				

Weekly Groceries for ____________________

NOTES

Weekly Meal Plan for ______________________

	BREAKFAST	LUNCH	DINNER	SNACKS
S				
M				
T				
W				
T				
F				
S				

Weekly Groceries for ____________________

- [ ] ______________________
- [ ] ______________________
- [ ] ______________________
- [ ] ______________________
- [ ] ______________________
- [ ] ______________________
- [ ] ______________________
- [ ] ______________________
- [ ] ______________________
- [ ] ______________________
- [ ] ______________________
- [ ] ______________________
- [ ] ______________________
- [ ] ______________________
- [ ] ______________________
- [ ] ______________________
- [ ] ______________________
- [ ] ______________________
- [ ] ______________________
- [ ] ______________________
- [ ] ______________________
- [ ] ______________________
- [ ] ______________________

- [ ] ______________________
- [ ] ______________________
- [ ] ______________________
- [ ] ______________________
- [ ] ______________________
- [ ] ______________________
- [ ] ______________________
- [ ] ______________________
- [ ] ______________________
- [ ] ______________________
- [ ] ______________________
- [ ] ______________________
- [ ] ______________________
- [ ] ______________________
- [ ] ______________________
- [ ] ______________________
- [ ] ______________________
- [ ] ______________________
- [ ] ______________________
- [ ] ______________________
- [ ] ______________________
- [ ] ______________________
- [ ] ______________________

NOTES

Weekly Meal Plan for ____________________

	BREAKFAST	LUNCH	DINNER	SNACKS
S				
M				
T				
W				
T				
F				
S				

Weekly Groceries for ____________________

NOTES

Weekly Meal Plan for ____________________

	BREAKFAST	LUNCH	DINNER	SNACKS
S				
M				
T				
W				
T				
F				
S				

Weekly Groceries for ______________________

NOTES

Weekly Meal Plan for ____________

	BREAKFAST	LUNCH	DINNER	SNACKS
S				
M				
T				
W				
T				
F				
S				

Weekly Groceries for ______________________

☐	______	☐	______
☐	______	☐	______
☐	______	☐	______
☐	______	☐	______
☐	______	☐	______
☐	______	☐	______
☐	______	☐	______
☐	______	☐	______
☐	______	☐	______
☐	______	☐	______
☐	______	☐	______
☐	______	☐	______
☐	______	☐	______
☐	______	☐	______
☐	______	☐	______
☐	______	☐	______
☐	______	☐	______
☐	______	☐	______
☐	______	☐	______
☐	______	☐	______
☐	______	☐	______
☐	______	☐	______
☐	______	☐	______

NOTES

Weekly Meal Plan for ____________________

	BREAKFAST	LUNCH	DINNER	SNACKS
S				
M				
T				
W				
T				
F				
S				

Weekly Groceries for ____________________

NOTES

Weekly Meal Plan for ______________________

	BREAKFAST	LUNCH	DINNER	SNACKS
S				
M				
T				
W				
T				
F				
S				

Weekly Groceries for ____________________

NOTES

Weekly Meal Plan for ________________

	BREAKFAST	LUNCH	DINNER	SNACKS
S				
M				
T				
W				
T				
F				
S				

Weekly Groceries for ______________

NOTES

Weekly Meal Plan for ____________________

	BREAKFAST	LUNCH	DINNER	SNACKS
S				
M				
T				
W				
T				
F				
S				

Weekly Groceries for ____________________

NOTES

Weekly Meal Plan for ____________________

	BREAKFAST	LUNCH	DINNER	SNACKS
S				
M				
T				
W				
T				
F				
S				

Weekly Groceries for ______________________

NOTES

Weekly Meal Plan for ____________________

	BREAKFAST	LUNCH	DINNER	SNACKS
S				
M				
T				
W				
T				
F				
S				

Weekly Groceries for ____________

NOTES

Weekly Meal Plan for ______________________

	BREAKFAST	LUNCH	DINNER	SNACKS
S				
M				
T				
W				
T				
F				
S				

Weekly Groceries for ____________

☐ ____________ ☐ ____________
☐ ____________ ☐ ____________
☐ ____________ ☐ ____________
☐ ____________ ☐ ____________
☐ ____________ ☐ ____________
☐ ____________ ☐ ____________
☐ ____________ ☐ ____________
☐ ____________ ☐ ____________
☐ ____________ ☐ ____________
☐ ____________ ☐ ____________
☐ ____________ ☐ ____________
☐ ____________ ☐ ____________
☐ ____________ ☐ ____________
☐ ____________ ☐ ____________
☐ ____________ ☐ ____________
☐ ____________ ☐ ____________
☐ ____________ ☐ ____________
☐ ____________ ☐ ____________
☐ ____________ ☐ ____________
☐ ____________ ☐ ____________
☐ ____________ ☐ ____________
☐ ____________ ☐ ____________
☐ ____________ ☐ ____________

NOTES

Weekly Meal Plan for ____________

	BREAKFAST	LUNCH	DINNER	SNACKS
S				
M				
T				
W				
T				
F				
S				

Weekly Groceries for ____________________

NOTES

Weekly Meal Plan for ____________________

	BREAKFAST	LUNCH	DINNER	SNACKS
S				
M				
T				
W				
T				
F				
S				

Weekly Groceries for ____________________

NOTES

Weekly Meal Plan for ____________________

	BREAKFAST	LUNCH	DINNER	SNACKS
S				
M				
T				
W				
T				
F				
S				

Weekly Groceries for ____________________

NOTES

Weekly Meal Plan for ______________________

	BREAKFAST	LUNCH	DINNER	SNACKS
S				
M				
T				
W				
T				
F				
S				

Weekly Groceries for ______________________

NOTES

Weekly Meal Plan for ____________________

	BREAKFAST	LUNCH	DINNER	SNACKS
S				
M				
T				
W				
T				
F				
S				

Weekly Groceries for ________________________

NOTES

Weekly Meal Plan for ____________________

	BREAKFAST	LUNCH	DINNER	SNACKS
S				
M				
T				
W				
T				
F				
S				

Weekly Groceries for ______________________

NOTES

Weekly Meal Plan for ____________________

	BREAKFAST	LUNCH	DINNER	SNACKS
S				
M				
T				
W				
T				
F				
S				

Weekly Groceries for ____________________

NOTES

Weekly Meal Plan for ____________

	BREAKFAST	LUNCH	DINNER	SNACKS
S				
M				
T				
W				
T				
F				
S				

Weekly Groceries for ____________________

NOTES

Weekly Meal Plan for ______________________

	BREAKFAST	LUNCH	DINNER	SNACKS
S				
M				
T				
W				
T				
F				
S				

Weekly Groceries for ____________________

NOTES

Made in the USA
Monee, IL
04 November 2026

67375612R00069